GASTROESOPHAGEAL REFLUX DISEASE

UNDERSTANDING EVERYTHING ABOUT GASTROESOPHAGEAL REFLUX DISEASE

DR. J. WALLER

Contents

INTRODUCTION

GERD, also referred to as gastroesophageal reflux disease, is a chronic illness that affects the digestive system. It happens when stomach contents or acid periodically runs back into the esophagus, causing discomfort and inflammation. Acid reflux is the term for this reflux of acid, which can result in a variety of symptoms and problems.

The muscular ring that divides the esophagus from the stomach, known as the lower esophageal sphincter (LES), typically acts as a valve to stop stomach contents from traveling back up into the esophagus. This valve weakens or relaxes in people with GERD, letting acid escape and irritating the lining of the esophagus.

Heartburn, regurgitation, chest pain, difficulty swallowing, and a persistent cough are all possible signs of GERD. Acid reflux is common, but frequent and prolonged episodes could be a sign of GERD. More serious side effects from GERD include esophagitis, Barrett's esophagus, and a higher chance of esophageal cancer if treatment is not received.

Medication, dietary adjustments, and lifestyle adjustments are frequently used to control GERD symptoms and avoid problems. Surgical procedures may be explored in cases that are more severe.

For those who are experiencing symptoms as well as the medical experts who are involved in their treatment, it is essential to comprehend GERD and how it is managed. Effective management options focus on symptom relief and overall digestive health improvement because the condition can have a major influence on quality of life.

CHAPTER ONE

What GERD Is

The chronic digestive ailment known as gastroesophageal reflux disease, or GERD, is typified by the reflux of stomach acid into the esophagus. The lower esophageal sphincter (LES), a muscular ring at the base of the esophagus, malfunctions to cause this condition, which is also referred to as acid reflux.

The LES weakens or relaxes improperly in people with GERD, which permits stomach contents including acid and occasionally bile to flow backward into the esophagus. When stomach acid is repeatedly exposed to the esophageal lining, it can cause irritation, inflammation, and other symptoms.

Principal Aspects of Gerd:

Acid Reflux: The regular and continuous reflux of stomach acid into the esophagus is the primary symptom of Gastrointestinal reflux disease (GERD).

Heartburn: One of the most prevalent signs of GERD is a burning feeling in the chest. It usually happens when you're lying down or after eating.

Regurgitation: GERD sufferers may feel as though food or acidic liquid is coming up into their mouths or throats from their stomachs.

Chest Pain: People with GERD may have discomfort or pain in the chest, which may prompt them to seek medical assistance if they have worries about heart problems.

Difficulty Swallowing: Also referred to as dysphagia, esophageal constriction (strictures) resulting in difficulty swallowing can happen in more advanced cases of GERD.

Chronic Cough: Stomach acid irritation of the airways is a common cause of persistent coughs, which can be worse by GERD.

Hoarseness and Laryngitis: When stomach acid refluxes into the throat, it can irritate the vocal cords, causing laryngitis and hoarseness.

Asthma problems: GERD can make breathing problems worse for people who have asthma.

Sleep Disturbances: Acid reflux can cause symptoms during the night, especially while sleeping down.

The diagnosis of GERD is made using a combination of the patient's symptoms, medical history, and results from diagnostic procedures such esophageal manometry, pH monitoring, and endoscopy. Lifestyle adjustments, dietary adjustments, drugs to lower acid production or increase esophageal motility, and in certain situations, surgical procedures are all part of the treatment plans for GERD.

It's critical to treat GERD as soon as possible because if left untreated or improperly managed, it can result in complications like Barrett's esophagus, esophagitis, and a higher risk of esophageal cancer. The goals of effective treatment for acid reflux are to reduce symptoms, enhance quality of life, and avoid long-term consequences.

Reasons and Initiators

The lower esophageal sphincter (LES), a muscle ring that serves as a valve between the esophagus and the stomach, is the primary cause of gastroesophageal reflux disease (GERD). The symptoms of GERD are brought on by the LES becoming weaker or relaxing, which permits stomach acid to reflux back into the esophagus. This dysfunction is caused by a number of reasons, and different triggers might make symptoms worse. The following are a few typical GERD causes and triggers:

Reasons:

The Lower Esophageal Sphincter (LES) is Weakened:

The main reason for GERD is a weak or malfunctioning LES. This may be brought on by variables like heredity, aging-related changes, and specific medical disorders.

Hiatal Hernia:

When a piece of the stomach pushes through the diaphragm into the chest, it can cause a hiatal hernia, which can interfere with the LES's ability to function and aggravate acid reflux.

Overweight:

Overweight puts more strain on the stomach and may be a factor in the LES's weakening, particularly around the abdomen.

Being pregnant:

Acid reflux may result from the pressure that the expanding uterus places on the stomach during pregnancy.

Disorders of Connective Tissue:

Scleroderma and other connective tissue disorders can alter how well the LES works.

Gastropteresis, or delayed emptying of the stomach:

Acid reflux can be exacerbated by illnesses like gastroparesis that slow down stomach emptying.

Triggers:

Specific Foods and Drinks:

GERD symptoms are frequently triggered by spicy or acidic foods, citrus fruits, tomatoes, chocolate, mint, caffeine, and alcoholic beverages.

Big or Heavy Meals:

Large or high-fat meals have the potential to relax the LES and raise the incidence of acid reflux.

Lying Down Following a Meal:

After eating, it may be easier for stomach acid to reflux back into the esophagus if you lie down or recline.

Smoking:

Smoking can increase acid production and decrease the LES, which increases a person's risk of developing GERD.

Tight Clothes:

Tight waistbands or belts can raise the pressure inside the abdomen, which may cause acid reflux.

Specific Drugs:

Certain pharmaceuticals, such as sedatives, calcium channel blockers, and several antihypertensive agents, have the potential to irritate the esophagus or relax the LES.

Posing a Lying or Bending Position:

Lying down or leaning over can be positions that increase the risk of acid reflux.

Stress

Although stress may not be the cause of GERD, it can make symptoms worse for those who already have it.

It's essential to comprehend the reasons and triggers of GERD in order to manage and avoid symptoms. Reducing the frequency and intensity of acid reflux episodes can be achieved by dietary changes, lifestyle improvements, and avoidance of identified triggers. People who have severe or ongoing GERD symptoms should contact a doctor for an appropriate diagnosis and treatment.

The symptoms of gastroesophageal reflux disease, or GERD, can range in severity from mild to severe. Stomach acid refluxing back into the esophagus is the main cause of GERD symptoms. Typical signs and symptoms include of:

Heartburn:

A common sign of GERD is a burning or uncomfortable feeling in the chest, frequently behind the breastbone. After eating or while you're sleeping, heartburn may get worse.

Recurrence:

Regurgitation is the feeling that stomach contents—such as acid or bile—are rising into the mouth or throat. There may be an aftertaste that is either bitter or sour.

Pain in the chest:

Chest discomfort brought on by GERD may resemble heart attack agony. It's critical to differentiate cardiac problems from GERD-related chest pain, and a medical checkup is advised.

Dysphagia, or difficulty swallowing:

GERD patients may experience dysphagia, which is persistent or recurrent difficulties swallowing. This may be the result of esophageal strictures, or narrowing.

Prolonged Cough:

GERD may be linked to a chronic cough that is unrelated to respiratory ailments like a cold or allergies. Stomach acid inflammation of the airways is a common cause of this cough.

Hoarseness and Laryngitis:

Stomach acid reflux into the throat can cause vocal cord inflammation, which can cause hoarseness and laryngitis.

Intolerance of Asthma:

Stomach acid reflux can make respiratory symptoms such as coughing and wheezing worse for those who have asthma.

CHAPTER TWO

Deterioration of Sleep Quality

GERD symptoms can cause sleep disturbances and nocturnal symptoms include regurgitation and coughing, especially while lying down.

emesis:

Some GERD sufferers may feel queasy, especially after eating or when they're lying down.

It's crucial to remember that not everyone with GERD has all of these symptoms, and that symptoms might vary in intensity. Furthermore, symptoms could be persistent or sporadic.

People should get evaluated by a doctor for accurate diagnosis and treatment if they think they may have GERD or if their symptoms are bothersome. Barrett's esophagus, esophagitis, and an elevated risk of esophageal cancer are among the problems that can arise from untreated or inadequately managed GERD.

Identification and Medical Assessment

In order to determine the degree of esophageal damage and establish the existence of acid reflux, diagnostic testing, clinical examination, and medical history assessment are all used in the diagnosis of gastroesophageal reflux disease (GERD). The following are essential elements of the GERD diagnosis and medical evaluation:

Health Background:

Getting a thorough medical history is the first step for healthcare professionals. This includes details about the frequency and intensity of symptoms, triggers, and any conditions that could make symptoms worse or better.

Evaluation of Symptoms:

An assessment of common GERD symptoms, including regurgitation, heartburn, chest pain, dysphagia, and persistent cough.

Physical Assessment:

In order to evaluate general health and find any indications or symptoms of GERD, a physical examination is performed. This could entail examining the abdomen and listening to the lungs.

Examine Acid-Suppressive Drugs:

In certain situations, medical professionals could advise trying acid-suppressive drugs, like proton pump inhibitors (PPIs) or H2 receptor blockers, to see if symptoms get better on their own. This may provide credence to the GERD diagnosis.

Endoscopy:

An endoscope, or flexible tube containing a camera, is inserted via the mouth and into the stomach and esophagus during an upper endoscopy operation. This enables the esophagus lining to be directly seen, any inflammation or damage to be identified, and, if necessary, the biopsy can be taken.

pH monitoring of the esophagus:

The acidity levels in the esophagus are measured over time via pH monitoring. It aids in determining the frequency and length of acid reflux episodes as well as their existence.

Gastric Manometry:

The strength and coordination of the esophageal muscles are measured by esophageal manometry. It assists in assessing the lower esophageal sphincter's (LES) performance and locating any anomalies in the motility of the esophagus.

Swallow Barium:

A barium swallow is ingesting a barium-containing contrast solution, which is then followed by X-ray imaging. This examination aids in the diagnosis of esophageal structural anomalies such hiatal hernias.

Testing for Impedance:

The assessment of gas and liquid movement in the esophagus is done using impedance testing. By giving more details regarding reflux occurrences, it can assist in the detection of non-acid reflux.

Esophageal Biopsy:

In the event that endoscopic findings reveal anomalies, tissue samples may be subjected to a biopsy in order to look for indications of

Barrett's esophagus, inflammation, or other disorders.

These diagnostic techniques work together to assist medical professionals in accurately diagnosing GERD, determining the severity of the illness, and identifying any complications or contributing factors. Following a diagnosis, the medical team might create a personalized treatment plan that includes lifestyle changes, medication, and, in certain situations, surgical procedures. In order to track the efficacy of the treatment plan and address any changes in symptoms or disease development, routine follow-up exams may be advised.

Treatment for Gastroesophageal reflux disease (GERD) consists of changing one's lifestyle, taking medicine, and sometimes undergoing surgery. Relieving symptoms, lowering the frequency of reflux episodes, and averting consequences are the objectives of treatment. The following are typical methods for treating GERD:

Changes in Lifestyle:

Dietary Adjustments: Steer clear of foods and drinks that set you off, such as chocolate, coffee, alcohol, and foods that are spicy, acidic, or fatty.

Meal timing: Avoiding large meals, especially right before bed, and opting instead for smaller, more frequent meals.

Weight management is the process of reaching and keeping a healthy weight in order to relieve stomach strain.

Posture and Sleeping Position: To prevent reflux throughout the night, avoid lying down or reclining after meals and raise the head of the bed.

Drugs:

Antacids: By neutralizing stomach acid, over-the-counter antacids can offer temporary relief.

H2 Receptor Blockers: Drugs like famotidine and ranitidine lessen the stomach's production of acid.

Proton Pump Inhibitors (PPIs): Often used for more severe cases, prescription or over-the-counter PPIs like omeprazole and esomeprazole reduce acid production more efficiently than H2 blockers.

Prokinetic Agents: These drugs, which include metoclopramide, improve stomach and esophageal motility and lower the risk of reflux.

Surgical Procedures:

Fundoplication: If medicine and lifestyle modifications don't work, surgery to implant a fundoplication may be a possibility. In order to strengthen the lower esophageal sphincter (LES), the upper part of the stomach is wrapped around the lower esophagus during this treatment.

LINX Device: To stop acid reflux while maintaining regular swallowing, a magnetic sphincter augmentation device, or LINX, can be implanted around the lower esophageal sphincter.

Endoscopic Procedures:

Endoscopic Radiofrequency Ablation (Stretta): This technique reduces reflux and strengthens the LES by using radiofrequency energy.

Endoscopic Suturing: To enhance the LES's functionality, sutures are placed endoscopically.

Esophageal Dilation Stretches:

When esophageal strictures arise, the narrowed portion of the esophagus can be widened by performing esophageal dilatation.

Weight Loss Surgery:

Bariatric surgery, or weight loss surgery, is a possibility for those with both GERD and obesity in order to treat both problems.

It's crucial to remember that treatment regimens are customized according to the degree of symptoms, whether problems exist, and how well early interventions work. It's critical to follow up with medical professionals on a regular basis to monitor symptoms, make any medication adjustments, and evaluate the efficacy of the selected course of therapy.

While many GERD sufferers find relief with conservative treatments and medications, those who experience severe or persistent symptoms, complications, or worry about taking medications over the long term should speak with healthcare providers to learn about the best course of action for their particular circumstances.

Changes in Lifestyle

In order to manage Gastroesophageal reflux disease (GERD) and lessen the frequency and intensity of reflux episodes, lifestyle changes are essential. Making the following lifestyle adjustments can help reduce symptoms and enhance digestive health in general:

Modifications to Diet:

Eat Less of Trigger Foods: Recognize and stay away from foods that make reflux worse, such as chocolate, coffee, alcohol, and spicy, acidic, and fatty meals.

Smaller, More Often Meals: Throughout the day, choose smaller, more frequent meals rather than larger, heavier ones.

When to Eat:

Avoid Eating Late at Night: Steer clear of heavy meals right before bed. Your last meal should be at least two or three hours before bed.

Eat Sitting Upright: To ease the strain on the stomach, sit up straight while eating.

Controlling Weight:

Retain a Healthy Weight: To lessen the chance of reflux and relieve stomach pressure, reach and maintain a healthy weight.

Sleeping position and posture:

Avoid Lying Down After Meals: After a meal, avoid reclining or lying down right away. To help with digestion, go for a leisurely walk instead.

Elevate the Head of the Bed: To stop reflux at night, raise the head of your bed by 6 to 8 inches by using bed risers or by putting blocks beneath the bedposts.

Options for Clothes:

Loose-Fitting Clothes: To prevent putting strain on the stomach, wear loose-fitting clothing, particularly around the waist.

Quitting Smoking:

Give Up Smoking: Smoking can cause acid reflux by weakening the lower esophageal sphincter (LES). Giving up smoking is good for managing GERD and general health.

Drinking Routines:

Remain Hydrated: To prevent severe stomach distension, drink liquids in between meals as opposed to during them.

Engaging in Exercise:

Regular Exercise: Take part in moderate exercise on a regular basis. Steer clear of intense exercise right after eating.

Handling Stress:

Relaxation Methods: Reduce stress, which can aggravate GERD symptoms, by practicing methods like deep breathing, yoga, or meditation.

Gum chewing:

Chew Sugar-Free Gum: Chewing gum increases salivation, which can lessen reflux and balance stomach acid.

Nutritional Modifications:

Alkaline Diet: Take into account including foods high in alkalinity, such as green vegetables, melons, and bananas, in your diet. These meals could aid in balancing gastric acid.

Spicy and Acidic Food Journal:

Maintain a Food Diary: Record your food decisions and any symptoms that arise. This can direct dietary adjustments and aid in the identification of particular triggers.

It's crucial to remember that everyone reacts differently to lifestyle changes. Even though many GERD sufferers find success with these adjustments, it's best to speak with a healthcare provider to develop a customized strategy that takes into account your unique symptoms and concerns. For best benefits, lifestyle changes should be constantly maintained in addition to medical therapies, as they are frequently utilized together.

Problems and Prolonged Handling

If long-term treatment for gastroesophageal reflux disease (GERD) is not successful, problems may result. Prolonged exposure of the esophagus to stomach acid can lead to complications, including inflammation and injury. The following are some possible side effects of untreated or inadequately controlled GERD along with long-term management techniques:

CHAPTER THREE

Problems:

esophagitis

The esophageal lining may become inflamed (esophagitis) as a result of repeated exposure to stomach acid. It could result in pain, discomfort, and trouble swallowing.

Barrett's Trachea:

Barrett's esophagus is a disorder where there are alterations in the cells lining the lower esophagus due to chronic GERD. This illness raises the chance of gastric cancer.

Restraints:

Scar tissue growth can cause the esophagus to narrow (strictures), which makes it harder for food to flow through.

Complicated Respiratory Systems:

Respiratory problems, such as pneumonia and persistent cough, can result from aspirating stomach contents into the lungs.

Extended-Term Administration:

Adherence to Medication:

following a doctor's prescription to take drugs to lower stomach acid production, such as H2 receptor blockers or proton pump inhibitors (PPIs).

Frequent Monitoring

routine follow-up visits with medical professionals to track symptoms, evaluate the efficacy of medications, and discuss any modifications to GERD treatment.

Changes in Lifestyle:

keeping up lifestyle adjustments, such as eating adjustments, weight control, and sleeping with the head of the bed raised, to reduce reflux attacks.

Endoscopic Monitoring:

Endoscopic surveillance may be advised for those with Barrett's esophagus in order to track the illness and spot any precancerous alterations.

Surgical Procedures:

When medicine and lifestyle changes are insufficient to relieve severe or chronic symptoms, surgical options including fundoplication or LINX device implantation may be explored.

Controlling Weight:

reaching and keeping a healthy weight in order to minimize pressure in the abdomen and lessen the likelihood of reflux.

Keeping Trigger Foods Away:

continuing to abstain from meals and drinks that can aggravate acid symptoms.

Continuous Stress Reduction:

managing stress, which can exacerbate GERD symptoms, by using stress-reduction strategies into daily living, such as mindfulness or relaxation activities.

Patient Instruction:

GERD sufferers should get continuing education regarding the disease, how to manage it, and the value of sticking to treatment regimens over the long term.

Examining for potential issues:

To evaluate how GERD is progressing and spot any issues early on, routine screenings and tests such as endoscopy and pH monitoring may be advised.

A thorough and customized strategy is needed for the long-term management of GERD in order to treat symptoms, avoid complications, and enhance general quality of life. To customize treatment programs based on individual needs and response to interventions, healthcare providers and GERD patients must work together. Follow-up and regular communication are crucial for effective long-term GERD management.

Useful Advice for GERD Patients

In order to successfully control symptoms, people with gastroesophageal reflux disease (GERD) must continuously pay attention to their lifestyle decisions and tactics. Here are some helpful hints for people who have GERD:

Nutritional Decisions:

Recognize and stay away from meals and drinks that can aggravate GERD symptoms. Acidic and spicy foods, chocolate, coffee, alcohol, and caffeine are common triggers.

To assist you in making educated dietary decisions, think about maintaining a food journal to record which foods might be connected to your symptoms.

Handling Meals:

Throughout the day, aim for smaller, more frequent meals as opposed to larger, heavier ones.

To lessen the chance of experiencing reflux at night, avoid eating right before bed. Your last meal should be at least two or three hours before bed.

Drinking Routines:

Drink liquids in between meals instead of during them to prevent undue distension of the stomach.

Sleeping position and posture:

When eating, keep your posture straight to ease the strain on your stomach.

To reduce reflux during the night, raise the head of your bed by 6 to 8 inches by using blocks or bed risers.

Controlling Weight:

A balanced diet and consistent exercise should be used to help you reach and stay at a healthy weight. Reflux and elevated intra-abdominal pressure can both be caused by excess weight.

Quitting Smoking:

Give up smoking since it can exacerbate GERD symptoms by weakening the lower esophageal sphincter (LES).

Handling Stress:

Utilize methods to reduce stress, including yoga, meditation, or deep breathing, as this might exacerbate the symptoms of GERD.

Options for Clothes:

Don loose-fitting garments, particularly those that fit around the waist, to prevent compressing the stomach.

Frequent Workout:

Exercise moderately and on a regular basis. Steer clear of intense exercise right after eating.

Gum chewing:

Chew on sugar-free gum to increase salivation, which can help counteract acid reflux.

Adherence to Medication:

Follow your doctor's instructions when taking prescription drugs, such as H2 receptor blockers or proton pump inhibitors (PPIs). For symptom control, drug regimen adherence is essential.

Frequent Monitoring

Make routine follow-up meetings with your physician to discuss treatment modifications, track your symptoms, and evaluate the efficacy of your drugs.

Examination and Endoscopy:

Undergo endoscopic screens or other testing as directed by your healthcare practitioner to keep an eye out for any issues, particularly if you have Barrett's esophagus.

Patient Instruction:

Keep yourself educated on GERD, its treatment, and any possible side effects. Learn the significance of following treatment regimens and changing one's lifestyle.

Assist Mechanism:

By talking to friends, relatives, or support groups about your experiences, you can create a network of support. Having a network of supporters can help one feel understood and encouraged.

Managing symptoms and averting consequences is a proactive, personalized strategy for living with GERD. You may reduce reflux episodes, improve general well-being, and live a more pleasant life with GERD by implementing these useful recommendations into your daily routine.

CONCLUSION

To sum up, Gastroesophageal reflux disease, or GERD, is a chronic illness that needs to be carefully managed and lifestyle changes made in order to reduce symptoms and avoid consequences. People with GERD can actively participate in their own well-being by learning about the causes and triggers of their condition and putting recommended daily living techniques into practice.

Due to the complex nature of GERD, a comprehensive strategy involving dietary adjustments, stress reduction, weight control, and, if required, medication or surgical procedures is required. Long-term management requires regular follow-up with healthcare practitioners, adherence to prescribed medicines, and awareness of potential consequences.

People with GERD can improve their quality of life by adopting lifestyle modifications, having a proactive mentality, and making educated dietary choices. Future improvements in outcomes are possible due to ongoing research and therapy choices that are evolving and adding to our understanding of GERD.

It is imperative that people with severe or chronic symptoms consult a medical expert for an accurate diagnosis and customized treatment regimens. People with GERD can overcome its hurdles and lead satisfying lives with well-managed symptoms if they have access to the appropriate techniques and a supportive healthcare team.

THE END